# A COMPREHENSIVE STUDY GUIDE ON STARTING PERIPHERAL IV'S

YOUR COMPLETE RESORCE GUIDE

# Vascular Access

## Welcome to Peripheral IV Insertion

CREATED BY
SHANE PENNINGTON, RN VA-BC

| CURRENT AS OF APRIL 2024 | | EDITED VERSION |

# Contents

✦

# Executive Summary

Hey there! Welcome to my guide on starting peripheral IVs. I'm thrilled to have you here, whether you're a healthcare professional looking to enhance your skills or simply a nursing student about to enter the world of intravenous therapy.

Now, you might be wondering why I am writing a study guide on this topic. Well, let me tell you a little bit about myself. I've spent the past three decades working as a PICC nurse in the healthcare field, and I've always been passionate about patient care. Over the years, I've gained extensive experience in starting peripheral IVs and have witnessed firsthand the impact it can have on patient outcomes.

I believe that knowledge should be shared, and that's why I've written this study guide. My goal is to provide you with a comprehensive resource that covers everything you need to know about starting peripheral IVs, from the anatomy and physiology behind it to the standards set by the Infusion Nurses Society.

So, whether you're a nursing student looking for a refresher, or a curious individual with a thirst for medical knowledge, I hope you find this book informative and helpful. Let's dive in and explore the fascinating world of peripheral IVs together.

*Let's begin...*

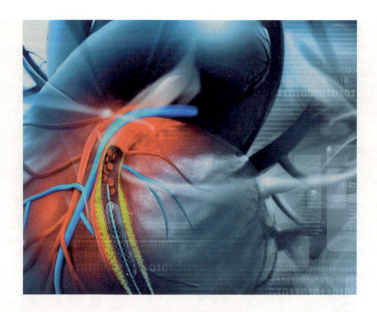

# About This Workbook

This study guide is designed to be a comprehensive resource for anyone interested in learning about starting peripheral IVs. Whether you are a beginner or a nursing student, this guide will provide you with the knowledge and skills necessary to safely and effectively perform this procedure.

Throughout the guide, you'll find detailed explanations of the anatomy and physiology of the peripheral veins, as well as step-by-step instructions on how to perform the procedure. I've also included tips and tricks that I've learned over the years to help make the process easier and less successful.

In addition to the practical aspects of starting peripheral IVs, this guide also covers the standards set by the Infusion Nurses Society. These standards are essential for ensuring patient safety and promoting best practices in intravenous therapy. By adhering to these standards, you'll be able to provide the highest level of care to your patients.

# How to Use This Study Guide

This study guide is organized into sections that cover different aspects of starting peripheral IVs. Each section builds upon the previous one, providing you with a logical and comprehensive learning experience.

I recommend starting with the section on anatomy and physiology, as it will provide you with a solid foundation of knowledge. Understanding the structure and function of the peripheral veins is crucial for performing the procedure effectively and minimizing the risk of complications.

Once you have a good grasp of the anatomy and physiology, you can move on to the section that covers the step-by-step process of starting a peripheral IV. This section will walk you through each stage of the procedure, from preparing the patient and gathering the necessary supplies to inserting the catheter and securing the line.

Finally, make sure to read the  complications, documentation and care and maintenance sections , these are essential for ensuring patient safety and providing quality care. Familiarize yourself with these guidelines to ensure that you are following best practices in intravenous therapy.

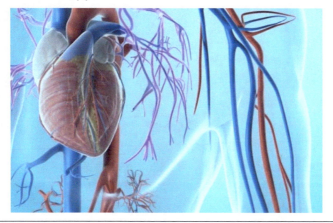

# Conclusion

Starting peripheral IVs is a crucial skill in healthcare, and I hope that this study guide will help you develop the knowledge and confidence to perform the procedure effectively. Remember, practice makes perfect, so don't be afraid to practice on simulation models or seek guidance from experienced professionals.
I'm excited for you to embark on this educational journey with me. Together, let's master the art of starting peripheral IVs and make a positive difference in the lives of our patients. Let's get started!

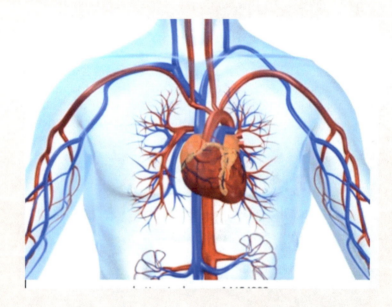

# Differences between Veins and Arteries

| Location | Vein: Superficial or deep |
| --- | --- |
| | Artery: Deep |
| Blood Flow | Vein: to the heart |
| | Artery: away from heart |
| Circulatory Function | Vein: numerous, supplied in networks, injury causes collateral vein use |
| | Artery: specific artery supplied by one vessel injury could result in tissue loss |
| Valves | Vein: valves |
| | Artery: no valves |
| Pulsation | Vein: no pulsation |
| | Artery: pulse can be felt as left ventricle contracts and pushes blood to aorta |
| Blood color | Vein: dark red, unoxygenated |
| | Artery: bright red due to oxygenation |

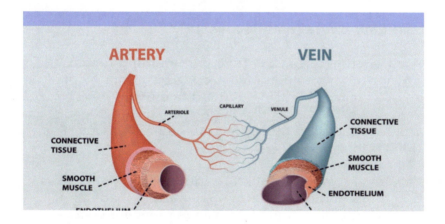

# Vessel (Vein) Anatomy

Vessel anatomy encompasses three distinct layers, each contributing to the structure and function of blood vessels:

## 1. Tunica Intima (inner layer):

Comprising a single layer of endothelial cells, the tunica intima forms the innermost lining of blood vessels.

In veins, this layer also plays a crucial role in the formation of valves, which help prevent backflow of blood and facilitate unidirectional flow towards the heart.

## 2. Tunica Media (middle layer):

Positioned between the tunica intima and tunica adventitia, the tunica media consists primarily of smooth muscle cells embedded in elastic fibers.

While thicker in arteries, the tunica media is relatively thinner in veins.

This layer is responsible for regulating vascular tone and diameter, allowing for vasodilation (widening) and vasoconstriction (narrowing) in response to physiological stimuli.

Additionally, the tunica media contains nerve fibers that contribute to the autonomic control of vascular function.

# Vessel (Vein) Anatomy

### 3. Tunica Adventitia (outer layer):

Composed predominantly of connective tissue, the tunica adventitia forms the outermost layer of blood vessels.

It is the thickest layer among the three tunics, providing structural support and stability to blood vessels.

The tunica adventitia also contains nerve fibers, blood vessels (vasa vasorum) that supply nutrients to the vessel wall, and lymphatic vessels.

Overall, the layered structure of blood vessels enables efficient blood flow regulation, maintenance of vascular integrity, and adaptation to changes in physiological conditions. The intricate interplay between these layers ensures proper functioning of the cardiovascular system, essential for maintaining homeostasis and overall health

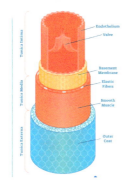 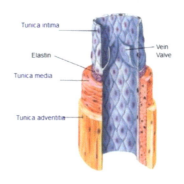

# Physiology

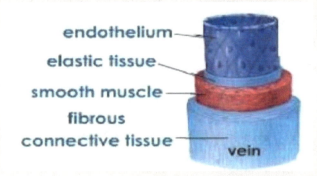

Understanding vessel anatomy is crucial for successful peripheral intravenous catheter (PIVC) insertion. Here are some key points to consider:

## 1. **Lack of Blood Return**

If you encounter a lack of blood return during PIVC insertion, it could indicate that the catheter tip is not properly positioned within the vein. It might be situated between the layers of the vein or adjacent to a valve, obstructing blood flow.

Proper technique and catheter selection are essential to minimize the risk of improper positioning and ensure adequate blood return.

# Physiology

### 2. **Catheter Length**

Using an appropriate catheter length is critical to ensure proper placement within the vein. Ideally, the catheter should be at least two-thirds (2/3) inside the vessel.

Catheters that are too short may rest against the vessel wall, increasing the risk of dislodgment, infiltration, or failure to maintain adequate blood flow.

Longer catheters provide better support and stability within the vein, reducing the likelihood of complications and improving catheter longevity.

By understanding the anatomy of blood vessels and adhering to best practices during PIVC insertion, healthcare providers can optimize patient outcomes and minimize the risk of complications.

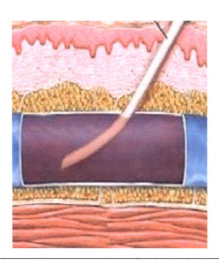

# STANDARDS OF PRACTICE

As a knowledgeable individual well-versed in medical standards, it's crucial to understand and adhere to established practices when performing procedures like peripheral intravenous catheter (PIVC) insertion. Here's an overview of some key standards:

### 1. Use the Smallest Gauge Catheter Possible in the Largest Vein

Selecting an appropriate catheter size is essential to minimize patient discomfort and reduce the risk of complications such as phlebitis or infiltration.

Using the smallest gauge catheter that meets the clinical requirements helps preserve vein integrity while ensuring adequate flow rates.

### 2. Ensure at Least 2/3 of the Catheter is in the Vein

Proper catheter placement within the vein is critical for optimal function and longevity.

Aim to insert the catheter so that at least two-thirds of its length resides within the vein, ensuring secure positioning and effective delivery of fluids or medications.

# STANDARDS OF PRACTICE

### 3. Choose the Vein Most Likely to Last the Full Length of Prescribed Therapy

Carefully assess the patient's veins to identify the most suitable site for catheter insertion.

Prioritize veins that are robust, accessible, and less prone to complications, considering factors such as vein size, visibility, and proximity to potential irritants.

### 4. Limit Insertion Attempts to Two per Clinician

Restricting the number of insertion attempts per clinician helps minimize patient discomfort, trauma to the veins, and the risk of complications.

If unsuccessful after two attempts, consider involving another qualified clinician or exploring alternative access options.

# STANDARDS OF PRACTICE

### 5. Consider Individual Patient Factors

Assess the patient's overall health status, vein condition, treatment duration, and medication requirements when planning PIVC insertion.

Take into account any contraindications or special considerations that may influence catheter selection and insertion technique.

Adhering to these standards of practice ensures safe and effective PIVC insertion, promotes patient comfort, and reduces the likelihood of complications, ultimately contributing to high-quality patient care.

# INDICATIONS

As a well-educated individual familiar with medical practices, it's important to understand the indications for peripheral intravenous (PIV) catheter insertion, particularly for short-term therapies. Here are the common indications for PIV placement:

## 1. Therapies for 4 days or less

PIV catheters are frequently utilized for short-term treatments, defined as therapies expected to last for four days or less. These may include various medical interventions that require intravenous access for a limited duration.

## 2. Hydration

PIV catheters are commonly inserted to provide hydration therapy, especially in cases of dehydration due to conditions such as vomiting, diarrhea, excessive sweating, or insufficient fluid intake.

Hydration via IV infusion helps replenish fluids, electrolytes, and essential nutrients quickly and effectively, restoring the body's hydration balance.

# INDICATIONS

### 3  Antibiotics and antivirals

PIV catheters are utilized for the administration of anti-infective medications, including antibiotics and antivirals, to treat bacterial, viral, fungal, or parasitic infections.

These medications may be given intravenously to achieve rapid and adequate drug concentrations, particularly in cases of severe or systemic infections where oral administration may be inadequate.

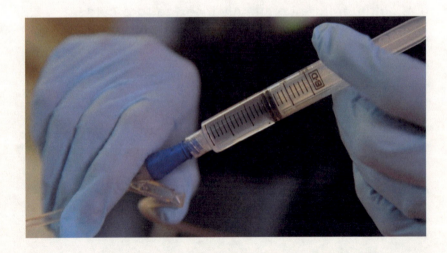

# INDICATIONS

## 4. IV Push Medications (Lasix, Solumedrol, or others per policy):

PIV catheters are employed for the delivery of medications via IV push or bolus administration, which involves administering a concentrated dose of medication directly into the bloodstream over a short duration.

Medications commonly administered via IV push include diuretics like Lasix (furosemide), corticosteroids like Solumedrol (methylprednisolone), and other drugs as determined by clinical protocols or institutional policies.

In summary, PIV catheters are indicated for a variety of short-term therapies, including hydration, administration of anti-infective medications, and IV push medications. Healthcare providers must assess the patient's condition, consider the therapeutic goals, and select the appropriate route of administration to ensure safe and effective treatment. Additionally, proper catheter care and monitoring are essential to prevent complications and promote optimal patient outcomes.

# CONTRAINDICATIONS

As an intelligent and well-educated individual, it's essential to grasp the contraindications for peripheral intravenous catheter (PIVC) placement to ensure patient safety and prevent potential complications. Here are the contraindications for PIVC placement:

### 1. Extremity with Dialysis Fistula or Shunt

Placing a PIVC in an extremity that houses a dialysis fistula or shunt is contraindicated to avoid damaging or obstructing these vital access points used for renal replacement therapy. Disruption of dialysis access can lead to complications such as thrombosis, infection, or inadequate dialysis.

### 2. Extremity with Recent Surgery

Avoiding extremities that have undergone recent surgical procedures is crucial to prevent disruption of surgical incisions, compromise healing, or introduce infection. Placing a PIVC in such extremities can increase the risk of wound dehiscence, infection, or impaired tissue healing.

AV Fistula

Artery
Vein
Blood from dialysis machine

Blood to dialysis machine

AV Fistula

Best choice for hemodialysis

Made by connecting an artery to a vein

Optimal blood flow

Lowest chance of infection

# CONTRAINDICATIONS

### 3. Extremity with Infections or Injury

PIVC placement is contraindicated in extremities with active infections, open wounds, or significant trauma. Inserting a catheter in these areas can introduce pathogens, exacerbate existing infections, or cause further tissue damage. It is essential to allow the affected extremity to heal adequately before considering PIVC placement.

### 4. Extremity Affected by Stroke or Decreased Sensation/Circulation

:
Extremities affected by conditions such as stroke, peripheral neuropathy, or compromised circulation present challenges for PIVC placement due to altered sensation, reduced blood flow, or impaired vascular integrity. Inserting a catheter in these extremities may be technically difficult and increase the risk of complications such as hematoma formation, tissue necrosis, or catheter-related thrombosis.

# CONTRAINDICATIONS

### 5. History of Breast Cancer or Lymph Node Resection

Extremities with a history of breast cancer or lymph node resection pose challenges for PIVC placement due to the risk of lymphedema, compromised lymphatic drainage, and potential impairment of venous circulation. Inserting a catheter in such extremities may exacerbate lymphedema or cause discomfort and compromise vascular access. Therefore, healthcare providers typically avoid placing PIVCs in extremities with a history of breast cancer or lymph node surgery.

### 6. History of Bilateral Breast Cancer

Patients with a history of bilateral breast cancer may have limited options for PIVC placement, especially if both upper extremities are affected by lymphedema or previous surgical interventions. In such cases, alternative sites for vascular access, such as the lower extremities or central venous access, may need to be considered.

# CONTRAINDICATIONS

## 7. Lymphedema:

While lymphedema is a contraindication for PIVC placement in extremities with a history of breast cancer or lymph node surgery, it's important to note that extremities without lymphedema may still be suitable for catheter insertion. Healthcare providers should carefully assess each patient's lymphatic status and vascular condition to determine the feasibility of PIVC placement.

## 8. Other Extremity Cannot Be Used

In some circumstances, the contralateral extremity may not be suitable for PIVC placement due to factors such as vascular access issues, previous interventions, or patient preference. When both upper extremities are not viable options for catheter insertion, healthcare providers may need to explore alternative sites or consider central venous access for vascular therapy.

# CONTRAINDICATIONS

Understanding these contraindications allows healthcare providers to make informed decisions regarding PIVC placement, ensuring patient safety and optimal outcomes. It's essential to assess each patient individually, considering their medical history, current condition, and anatomical factors before proceeding with PIVC insertion.

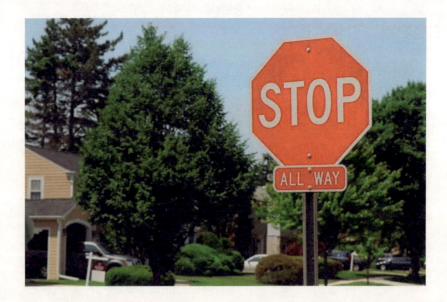

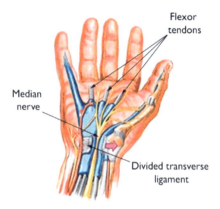

Median nerve — Flexor tendons — Divided transverse ligament

# Potiential for nerve damage

It  is important to recognize the potential for nerve damage during the process of starting a peripheral intravenous (PIV) line. Here are some key points to consider:

### 1. Avoiding Placement on the Inside of the Wrist

The inside of the wrist contains delicate nerves and structures that can be easily damaged during PIV insertion. Nerve damage in this area can lead to significant pain, tingling, numbness, or even loss of function in the hand and fingers. Therefore, healthcare providers should refrain from placing PIVs on the inner wrist to prevent nerve injury and its associated complications.

# Potiential for nerve damage

### 2. **Exercise Caution with Outer Wrist Placement**

If it becomes necessary to insert a PIV in the outer wrist area, healthcare providers should exercise caution to avoid damaging the radial nerve. This nerve runs along the outer aspect of the wrist and is susceptible to injury during catheter placement. To minimize the risk of nerve damage, it's advisable to position the catheter at least two fingers' width above the wrist bend, where the radial nerve is less likely to be affected.

### 3. **Prompt Response to Patient Complaints**:

Patients should be closely monitored during and after PIV insertion for any signs or symptoms of nerve damage, such as pain or tingling in the wrist or hand. If a patient experiences discomfort or neurological symptoms, the PIV should be removed immediately to prevent further nerve injury. Timely intervention is crucial to minimizing the impact of nerve damage and ensuring patient safety and well-being.

By being aware of the potential for nerve damage during PIV insertion and taking appropriate precautions, healthcare providers can mitigate the risk of complications and promote optimal outcomes for patients. Prioritizing patient safety and comfort is essential in all aspects of clinical practice, including vascular access procedures like PIV insertion.

# INSERTION PROCEDURE

# PREPARATION

As someone who values knowledge and education, it's crucial to grasp the intricacies of peripheral intravenous (PIV) insertion, a routine medical procedure employed to deliver fluids, medications, or therapies directly into a patient's vein. Let's delve into the detailed process of PIV insertion:

1. **Verify MD Order:**

Before initiating the procedure, ensure that there is a valid physician's order authorizing the insertion of the PIV.

2. **Gather Supplies:**

Collect all the necessary supplies for the PIV insertion procedure. This typically includes an IV start kit, an IV catheter, extension tubing, and a normal saline flush.

3. **Explain Procedure to Patient/Obtain Consent**

Communicate with the patient to explain the purpose and process of the PIV insertion. Obtain informed consent from the patient, ensuring they understand the procedure and its potential risks and benefits.

# INSERTION PROCEDURE

# PREPARATION

### 4. Prepare Workspace

Set up a clean and organized workspace conducive to performing the PIV insertion procedure safely and efficiently.

### 5. Open IV Start Kit and Supplies

Open the IV start kit and arrange the supplies in a convenient manner for easy access during the procedure.

By following these initial steps, healthcare providers can ensure that the PIV insertion procedure is conducted in a systematic and patient-centered manner, prioritizing safety, efficacy, and patient communication.

Let's do this!

# INSERTION PROCEDURE

# SITE SELECTION

To initiate the process of peripheral intravenous (PIV) insertion, first, ensure proper hand hygiene is performed. Next, position the patient comfortably for the procedure. Apply a tourniquet to the patient's arm to aid in vein visualization and assessment. Once the vein is identified, remove the tourniquet. Then, prepare the IV extension tubing by priming it with Normal Saline solution to facilitate smooth insertion and subsequent medication delivery.

# INSERTION PROCEDURE

# EVALUATION

To begin the peripheral intravenous (PIV) insertion process, start by assessing the patient's veins using a tourniquet. Once a suitable site is found, remove the tourniquet. Encourage the patient to make a fist a few times to help dilate the veins and make them more visible and accessible.

To further enhance vein dilation and improve insertion success, apply warm moist packs to the selected site. This can be achieved by using a towel moistened with warm water and covering it with plastic wrap or a clean trash bag. Alternatively, a clean glove can be filled with warm water, tied securely, and placed on the extremity. It is crucial to ensure that the temperature of the water is comfortable for the patient and will not cause any burns.

By following these steps, you can optimize vein visibility and make the PIV insertion process more comfortable and successful for the patient.

# INSERTION PROCEDURE

# EVALUATION

To facilitate the peripheral intravenous (PIV) insertion process, it's essential to utilize gravity effectively. Position the patient in such a way that allows gravity to assist in vein dilation and blood flow.

If the patient is sitting or lying on a bed, let the extremity where the PIV will be inserted hang down off the side of the bed. This positioning encourages blood flow to the veins in the arm, making them more prominent and easier to access.

If the patient is lying flat in bed, consider raising the head of the bed slightly if possible. Elevating the head of the bed can help promote venous return and enhance the visibility and accessibility of the veins in the arm.

By optimizing the positioning of the patient and utilizing gravity, you can improve the success rate of PIV insertion and enhance the overall patient experience.

# INSERTION PROCEDURE

To begin the process of peripheral intravenous (PIV) insertion, it's crucial to prepare the designated insertion site meticulously. Here's a step-by-step guide:

1. **Prep designated site using appropriate antimicrobial:**

Choose an appropriate antimicrobial solution such as chlorhexidine/alcohol. This solution effectively disinfects the skin and reduces the risk of infection.

2. **Cleanse site with gentle scrubbing motion:**

Apply the antimicrobial solution to the designated insertion site and cleanse the area using a gentle scrubbing motion. Ensure thorough coverage of the skin to eliminate any potential pathogens.

3. **No Shaving!! Clip hair if necessary:**

Avoid shaving the insertion site as it can increase the risk of skin irritation and infection. Instead, if there is excessive hair present, use clippers to trim the hair short without removing it entirely.

# INSERTION PROCEDURE

### 4. . Apply tourniquet:

Once the site is cleansed andprepared, apply a tourniquet proximal to the insertion site. The tourniquet helps distend the veins, making them more visible and accessible for insertion.

### 5. Don gloves in kit or clean gloves if not in kit:

Prior to initiating the insertion procedure, don gloves from the IV start kit or clean gloves if they are not included in the kit. Wearing gloves ensures proper infection control and protects both the patient and the healthcare provider.

### 6. Stabilize vein by applying traction to skin:

Gently pull the skin taut in the direction of the vein to stabilize it. This helps to prevent the vein from rolling and facilitates easier insertion of the catheter.

### 7. Do not palpate vein again:

Once the vein is stabilized, avoid palpating it again to minimize the risk of vein collapse or injury

# INSERTION PROCEDURE

8. **Bevel Position:**

Hold catheter by flash chamber with needle bevel side up over vein in direction of blood flow. Hold the catheter firmly by the flash chamber, ensuring that the needle bevel is facing upward. Position the catheter directly over the vein in the direction of the blood flow.

9. **Insert catheter through skin and vein observing for flashback:**

Insert the catheter through the skin and into the vein while closely observing for flashback. Flashback is the indication that the catheter tip has entered the vein and blood is flowing into the catheter hub.

For superficial veins, insert the catheter at a 15-degree angle.

For deeper veins, insert the catheter at a 25-30-degree angle.

10. **When flashback is noted,**

lower catheter until almost flush with skin and advance so stylet and catheter are in the vein:** Once you observe flashback, indicating that the catheter is successfully inserted into the vein, gently lower the catheter until it is nearly flush with the skin. Then, advance the catheter further into the vein to ensure that both the stylet and catheter are completely within the vein.

# INSERTION PROCEDURE

## 11. Advance catheter:

Only, off the stylet until the entire catheter is inserted up to the hub:** After ensuring that both the stylet and catheter are in the vein, continue to advance the catheter further into the vein while withdrawing the stylet. This ensures that the entire length of the catheter is inserted into the vein up to the hub.

## 12. Depending upon the type of catheter, it may be necessary to apply digital pressure prior to retracting the needle

In some cases, especially with smaller gauge catheters or fragile veins, it may be necessary to apply gentle digital pressure near the insertion site before retracting the needle. This helps to stabilize the catheter and prevent it from dislodging during needle removal.

## 13. Release tourniquet:

Once the catheter is securely in place and the needle is retracted, release the tourniquet from the patient's arm. This allows normal blood flow to resume in the vein.

# INSERTION PROCEDURE

### 14. Retract stylet:

Finally, retract the stylet completely from the catheter. Ensure that the stylet is fully removed and disposed of properly.

### 15. Attach primed extension to hub of catheter:

Once the catheter is securely in place, attach the primed extension tubing to the hub of the catheter. This extension tubing allows for the administration of fluids or medications through the catheter.

### 16. Apply transparent dressing to cover site taping securely to minimize movement or dislodgement:

After attaching the extension tubing, apply a transparent dressing over the insertion site. The dressing should be applied securely but not too tight to avoid restricting blood flow. The transparent dressing helps to protect the site from contamination and minimizes movement or dislodgement of the catheter.

# INSERTION PROCEDURE

**17. Flush catheter with remaining 0.9% NS and check again for blood return:**

Finally, flush the catheter with the remaining 0.9% normal saline (NS) solution to ensure that it is patent and functioning properly. After flushing, check again for blood return to confirm proper placement of the catheter within the vein. If there is no blood return or if there are any signs of complications, such as swelling or discomfort at the insertion site, further assessment and intervention may be necessary.

18: **Apply tape to secure extension set:**

Once the extension set is attached to the hub of the catheter and the dressing is in place, secure the extension set with tape. This helps to prevent accidental dislodgement or movement of the catheter during patient care activities.

19: **Remove gloves:**

After securing the extension set, carefully remove the gloves used during the procedure. Proper glove removal technique is important to avoid contaminating hands or other surfaces.

# INSERTION PROCEDURE

20: **Perform hand hygiene:**

Following glove removal, perform hand hygiene using soap and water or alcohol-based hand sanitizer. Hand hygiene is essential to prevent the spread of infection and maintain a sterile environment during patient care.

20. **Document:**

Finally, document the PIV insertion procedure in the patient's medical record. Document important details such as the date and time of insertion, site location, catheter size, any complications encountered, and patient response. Accurate documentation ensures continuity of care and provides valuable information for other healthcare providers involved in the patient's treatment.

By completing these final steps, you ensure that the PIV insertion procedure is conducted safely and effectively, with proper attention to infection control and documentation practices.

# DOCUMENTATION

Certainly! Here's an explanation of the final documentation steps in the PIV insertion process:

1. **Exact site:**

Document the precise location where the PIV was inserted on the patient's body. This includes noting the specific vein used and any anatomical landmarks that may aid in future assessments or interventions.

2. **Gauge and length of catheter:**

Record the size (gauge) and length of the catheter used for the PIV insertion. This information is crucial for monitoring the adequacy of the catheter for the patient's needs and for selecting appropriate infusion devices.

3. **Number of attempts:**

Document the number of attempts made by each healthcare provider involved in the PIV insertion. Typically, healthcare professionals are limited to two attempts per insertion, and only two nurses should be involved in the process to minimize patient discomfort and risk of complications.

# DOCUMENTATION

### 4. **Blood return:**

Note whether blood return was observed after catheter insertion. Blood return indicates successful placement of the catheter within the vein and ensures proper functionality for medication administration and fluid therapy.

### 5. **Additional Devices:**

Document any additional devices or attachments connected to the PIV, such as extension tubing, infusion pumps, or syringe ports. This information helps to ensure proper monitoring and management of the PIV site throughout the patient's care.

### 6 **Flush:**

Document the process of flushing the PIV catheter with saline solution after insertion. This includes recording the volume of saline used for flushing and any observations related to the flush, such as ease of flow or resistance encountered. Documenting the flush ensures that the catheter is patent and ready for medication administration or fluid therapy.

# DOCUMENTATION

### 7. Dressing:

Record details about the dressing applied to the PIV insertion site. Document the type of dressing used (e.g., transparent film, gauze and tape) and its adherence to infection control protocols. Note any specific instructions provided for dressing care and maintenance, such as frequency of dressing changes or signs of infection to monitor.

### 8. Patient tolerance:

Document the patient's response to the PIV insertion procedure, including their level of discomfort, pain, or anxiety. Use a standardized pain assessment scale, if available, to quantify the patient's pain intensity. Note any interventions implemented to address discomfort, such as administration of local anesthetic or repositioning for comfort.

### 9. Patient education, potential barriers:

Document any patient education provided regarding the PIV insertion procedure, care of the PIV site, and signs of complications to monitor for. Note any barriers to effective patient education, such as language barriers, cognitive impairments, or limited health literacy, and document strategies employed to overcome these barriers, such as using visual aids or involving family members as interpreters.

# DOCUMENTATION

By documenting these aspects of the PIV insertion process, healthcare providers can ensure comprehensive and accurate documentation of patient care, facilitate communication among members of the healthcare team, and promote patient safety and satisfaction.

# COMPLICATIONS
# PHLEBITIS

Here's an explanation of complications associated with peripheral intravenous (PIV) catheter insertion.

**Mechanical Phlebitis:**

1. **Catheter too big:**

Using a catheter that is too large for the size of the vein can lead to mechanical complications such as vein trauma, increased risk of infiltration, and discomfort for the patient.

2. **Area of flexion allows catheter to piston in and out with movement:**

Placing the PIV catheter in an area prone to frequent movement, such as near joints or on the hands, can cause the catheter to piston in and out with patient movement. This mechanical stress increases the risk of catheter dislodgement, infiltration, or phlebitis.

3. **Improper stabilization of catheter:**

Failing to adequately secure the PIV catheter to the patient's skin can result in catheter movement or dislodgement, increasing the risk of complications such as infiltration, infection, or accidental removal.

# COMPLICATIONS
# PHLEBITIS

**Chemical Phlebitis:**

1. **Irritated or vesicant-infused medications:**

Administering irritating or vesicant medications through a PIV catheter can lead to chemical irritation, tissue necrosis, or extravasation injury. Vesicant medications have the potential to cause severe tissue damage if they infiltrate surrounding tissues.

2. **Improperly diluted medications:**

Administering medications that are improperly diluted or prepared can result in chemical irritation or adverse drug reactions. Incorrect dilution can lead to osmotic imbalances, phlebitis, or thrombophlebitis.
3. **Giving medication too fast:** Rapid infusion of medications through a PIV catheter can overwhelm the vein, causing venous irritation, phlebitis, or infiltration. It can also increase the risk of adverse drug reactions or systemic complications.

Understanding these potential complications is crucial for healthcare providers to mitigate risks, ensure patient safety, and provide high-quality care during PIV catheter insertion and medication administration. Proper assessment, monitoring, and adherence to best practices can help prevent or minimize these complications in clinical practice.

# COMPLICATIONS
# INFILTRATION

Here's an explanation of infiltration complications associated with peripheral intravenous (PIV) catheter insertion.

**Signs and Symptoms**:

1. **Cool:**

The affected area may feel cooler than the surrounding skin due to impaired blood flow caused by infiltration of fluids or medications into the surrounding tissues.

2. **Blanched:**

The skin around the PIV site may appear pale or whitened, indicating compromised blood flow and potential tissue damage due to the accumulation of fluid.

3. **Swollen:**

Swelling at or around the PIV site is a common sign of infiltration, indicating the accumulation of fluids in the surrounding tissues.

# COMPLICATIONS
# INFILTRATION

4. **Tender or painful:**

Patients may experience tenderness or pain at the PIV site, which can result from tissue irritation, inflammation, or pressure caused by the infiltrated fluid.

5. **Leaking at the site:**

Leakage of fluid or medication from the PIV site suggests infiltration, where the infused solution enters the surrounding tissues instead of the vein.

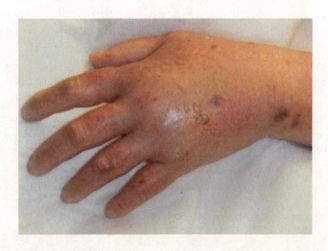

# COMPLICATIONS
# INFILTRATION

**Treatment:**

### 1. Remove PIVC:

Prompt removal of the PIV catheter is essential to prevent further infiltration and minimize tissue damage. This involves gently withdrawing the catheter from the insertion site.

### 2. Elevate extremity:

Elevating the affected extremity above the level of the heart helps reduce swelling and promote venous return, aiding in the resolution of infiltration.

### 3. Warm compresses:

Applying warm compresses to the affected area can help improve blood circulation, reduce discomfort, and promote tissue healing. Warmth also helps alleviate symptoms such as pain and swelling by increasing tissue perfusion.

Understanding these signs, symptoms, and treatment options is crucial for healthcare providers to promptly recognize and manage infiltration complications associated with PIV catheter insertion. By taking appropriate action, providers can mitigate risks, optimize patient outcomes, and ensure safe and effective care delivery.

# COMPLICATIONS
# SITE INFECTION

it's essential to understand the complications associated with site infections following peripheral intravenous (PIV) catheter insertion:

**Complications:**

1. **Due to Poor Insertion Technique:**

Infections can occur at the PIV site due to inadequate sterile technique during catheter insertion. If proper aseptic precautions are not followed, microorganisms from the skin or environment may contaminate the insertion site, leading to infection.

2. **Poor Dressing Maintenance:**

Inadequate or improper dressing maintenance can increase the risk of site infections. Failure to regularly monitor and change the dressing, as well as improper securing of the dressing, can compromise the integrity of the insertion site, allowing pathogens to enter and cause infection.

# COMPLICATIONS
# SITE INFECTION

## Signs and Symptoms of Infection:

- Redness or erythema around the PIV site
- Swelling or edema
- Increased warmth or localized heat at the site
- Pain or tenderness
- Purulent drainage or discharge
- Fever or systemic signs of infection (severe cases)

## Preventive Measures:

### 1. Proper Insertion Technique:

Ensuring adherence to strict aseptic technique during PIV catheter insertion is crucial to prevent site infections. This includes thorough hand hygiene, use of sterile gloves and equipment, and meticulous site preparation.

### 2. Dressing Care:

Regular assessment and maintenance of the PIV site dressing are essential to prevent infections. Dressings should be changed according to facility protocols or when visibly soiled, and proper technique should be employed to ensure a snug and secure fit.

# COMPLICATIONS
# SITE INFECTION

**Management:**

Early detection and prompt management of site infections are essential to prevent complications and promote healing. Treatment typically involves removing the infected catheter, initiating appropriate antimicrobial therapy if necessary, and implementing wound care measures.

Understanding these complications and their preventive measures is vital for healthcare providers to ensure safe and effective PIV catheter insertion and minimize the risk of site infections in patients. By adhering to best practices and maintaining vigilance, providers can contribute to better patient outcomes and reduce the incidence of complications associated with PIV catheterization.

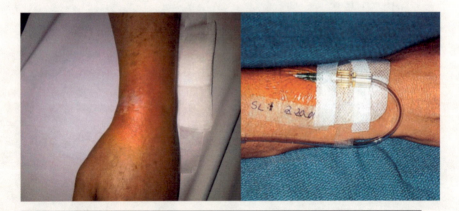

# COMPLICATIONS
# EXTRAVASATION

it's important to recognize the complications associated with extravasation during peripheral intravenous (IV) therapy:

**Extravasation of Irritant or Vesicant Medications:**

Extravasation occurs when irritant or vesicant medications intended for intravenous administration leak out of the vein and into the surrounding tissue. Irritant medications may cause discomfort and inflammation, while vesicants have the potential to cause severe tissue damage, blistering, or necrosis.

**Signs and Symptoms:**

1.**Complaints of Pain or Burning:**

Patients may experience localized pain or a burning sensation at the IV site or along the path of extravasation.

2.**Swelling Around IV Site**:

Extravasation can lead to tissue swelling and edema around the IV insertion site, indicating infiltration of fluid or medication into the surrounding tissues.

# COMPLICATIONS
# EXTRAVASATION

### 3.IV Not Running or Alarming Occlusion:

A sudden cessation of IV flow or an occlusion alarm from the infusion pump may indicate extravasation, especially if accompanied by swelling or pain at the site.

### Management:

### 1.Immediate Action:

Upon suspicion or confirmation of extravasation, it's essential to take immediate action to minimize tissue damage and mitigate patient discomfort. Stop the infusion immediately to prevent further medication infiltration.

### 2.Elevation:

Elevating the affected limb above the level of the heart can help reduce swelling and minimize the spread of the extravasated medication.

### 3.Warm Compresses:

Application of warm compresses to the affected area can help promote vasodilation, improve blood flow, and facilitate the absorption and dispersion of the extravasated medication.

_ *

# COMPLICATIONS
# EXTRAVASATION

## 4.Referral and Treatment:

Depending on the severity of the extravasation and the nature of the medication involved, patients may require further assessment and treatment. Some cases may necessitate consultation with a pharmacist or specialist for specific antidotes or interventions.

## Documentation and Follow-Up:

### 1.Documentation:

It's important to document the extravasation event thoroughly, including the type and volume of medication involved, the signs and symptoms observed, and the actions taken in response.

### 2. Follow-Up:

Patients should be closely monitored for signs of tissue damage or complications following extravasation. Follow-up assessments may be required to evaluate the resolution of symptoms and ensure adequate wound healing.

# COMPLICATIONS
# EXTRAVASATION

By recognizing the signs and symptoms of extravasation and taking prompt and appropriate action, healthcare providers can minimize the potential for tissue injury and promote optimal patient outcomes during IV therapy. Additionally, adherence to facility policies and guidelines is essential for standardizing management practices and ensuring patient safety.

# COMPLICATIONS
# EXTRAVASATION PICTURES

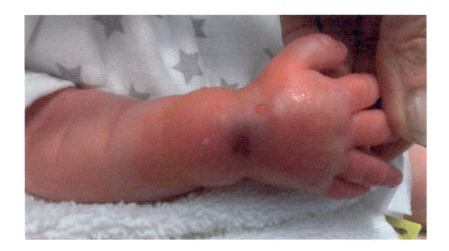

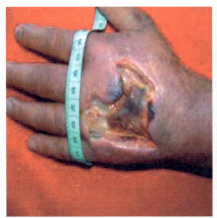

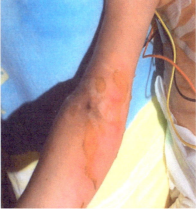

# CARE AND MAINTENANCE

It is crucial to understand the care and maintenance protocols for peripheral intravenous catheters (PIVCs) to ensure optimal patient outcomes. Here are some general instructions, although it's important to always refer to your facility's policy for specific guidelines:

**Care and Maintenance of PIV:**

1. **Assessment Frequency:**

Assess the PIVC site every 4 hours as part of routine nursing care.

Increase the assessment frequency to every 2 hours for patients who are critically ill, sedated, or have cognitive deficits.

2. **Change PIVC Site:**

Change the PIVC site only when clinically indicated, such as:

Redness, swelling, or tenderness at the insertion site.

Occlusion of the catheter, impeding infusion flow.

Consider changing the PIVC site within 24 hours if it was inserted at an outside facility or by emergency medical services (EMS) to minimize the risk of infection.

# CARE AND MAINTENANCE

### 3. Flush Protocol:

Flush the PIVC every 8 hours with at least 3 mL of normal saline (NS) if the catheter is not actively in use.

After administering medication or blood products through the PIVC, flush the catheter with no less than 5 mL of NS to ensure adequate medication delivery and prevent catheter occlusion.

### Additional Considerations:

### 1. Documentation:

Document all PIVC assessments, flushes, and any changes in the patient's condition or the PIVC site in the medical record according to facility guidelines.

### 2. Patient Education:

Educate patients about the importance of reporting any discomfort, swelling, or changes at the PIVC site promptly. Encourage patients to notify healthcare providers if they experience any signs of infection or complications.

# CARE AND MAINTENANCE

### 3. Infection Prevention:

Follow strict aseptic technique during PIVC care and maintenance to reduce the risk of infection. Ensure proper hand hygiene and use appropriate personal protective equipment when handling PIVCs.

### 4. Collaboration:

Collaborate with other healthcare team members, such as nurses, physicians, and infusion therapy specialists, to address any concerns or complications related to PIVCs promptly.

By adhering to these care and maintenance practices, healthcare providers can help minimize the risk of complications associated with PIVCs and promote patient safety and comfort during intravenous therapy.

# INFUSION NURSES SOCIETY (INS) STANDARDS

The Infusion Nurses Society Infusion Therapy Standards of Practice (INS Standards) is a comprehensive set of guidelines that serve as the gold standard for infusion therapy practices in healthcare facilities. Developed by the Infusion Nurses Society (INS), these standards are based on the latest evidence-based research and aim to standardize and improve the quality of intravenous (IV) therapy delivery across various healthcare settings.

It's important to understand the significance of these standards in ensuring the safety and efficacy of IV therapy. The INS Standards cover a wide range of topics related to infusion therapy, including but not limited to:

1. **Patient Assessment:**

Guidelines for assessing patients' vascular access needs, including vein selection, assessing for complications, and determining appropriate device selection.

# INFUSION NURSES SOCIETY (INS) STANDARDS

### 2. Vascular Access Device Selection and Management:

Recommendations for selecting the most appropriate vascular access device based on patient-specific factors, as well as guidelines for device insertion, maintenance, and removal.

### 3. Infection Prevention:

Protocols for preventing infections associated with IV therapy, including recommendations for hand hygiene, aseptic technique during device insertion, and catheter site care.

### 4. Documentation and Quality Improvement:
Standards for documenting infusion therapy procedures and patient responses, as well as guidelines for quality improvement initiatives to enhance patient outcomes.

### 5. Complications Management:

Strategies for identifying and managing complications related to infusion therapy, such as catheter-related bloodstream infections, infiltration, extravasation, and phlebitis.

# INFUSION NURSES SOCIETY (INS) STANDARDS

By adhering to the INS Standards, healthcare facilities can ensure consistency and excellence in the delivery of infusion therapy services, ultimately leading to improved patient outcomes, reduced complications, and enhanced patient satisfaction. As a healthcare professional, it's essential to familiarize yourself with these standards and incorporate them into your practice to provide safe and effective care to your patients.

## Appropriate Catheter Size

it's crucial to understand the significance of the Infusion Nurses Society (INS) standards in guiding the practice of infusion therapy. One key aspect emphasized by the INS Standards is the selection of appropriate catheter size for peripheral intravenous catheters (PIVC).

According to the INS Standards, it is recommended to use the smallest-gauge PIVC that can adequately accommodate the prescribed therapy and meet the patient's needs. This recommendation is based on evidence-based research and aims to minimize patient discomfort, reduce the risk of complications, and optimize the effectiveness of IV therapy.

# INFUSION NURSES SOCIETY (INS) STANDARDS

Furthermore, the INS Standards highlight the importance of utilizing vascular visualization technology, such as ultrasound or infrared devices, to enhance the success rate of PIVC insertion, particularly in patients with difficult intravenous access (DIVA). These technologies can assist healthcare providers in identifying suitable veins for catheter insertion, improving first-attempt success rates, and reducing the incidence of insertion-related complications.

Additionally, maintaining the recommended catheter-to-vessel ratio is essential to ensure proper blood flow and prevent vein damage or thrombosis. Adhering to these standards helps healthcare professionals deliver safe and effective infusion therapy, ultimately contributing to better patient outcomes and satisfaction.

By integrating the INS Standards into clinical practice, healthcare providers can uphold the highest quality of care and ensure optimal outcomes for patients receiving IV therapy. As a well-educated individual, it's imperative to stay informed about these standards and implement them in daily practice to promote excellence in infusion therapy delivery.

# INFUSION NURSES SOCIETY (INS) STANDARDS

## Site Selection

The INS standards emphasize the importance of selecting the appropriate site for intravenous (IV) insertion, with a focus on preserving vessel health and minimizing potential complications.

When selecting the site for IV insertion, it's essential to consider the proposed treatment plan. This means understanding the specific needs of the patient and the type of medication or fluid being administered. Additionally, the overall health of the patient's veins should be taken into account. Vein preservation is a key aspect, as repeated punctures can lead to vein damage and decreased access in the future.

Collaboration is emphasized between the healthcare team and the patient, as well as their family or caregivers. This collaborative approach ensures that all stakeholders are involved in the decision-making process. Patients and their caregivers may have valuable insights into their medical history, previous experiences with IV therapy, and personal preferences that can inform site selection.

# INFUSION NURSES SOCIETY (INS) STANDARDS

By adhering to these standards, healthcare professionals can ensure that IV insertion is performed with precision and consideration for the patient's well-being. This not only improves the overall quality of care but also minimizes the risks associated with IV therapy.

**Site Prep**

The INS (Infusion Nurses Society) standards regarding disinfection is vital for ensuring patient safety and preventing infections during vascular access procedures.

The INS standards emphasize the importance of proper hand hygiene as a fundamental step before inserting an IV catheter. This practice helps reduce the risk of transferring harmful microorganisms from the hands of healthcare professionals to the patient's bloodstream.

Before placing a vascular access device, skin antisepsis is essential. This involves cleaning the puncture site to eliminate any microorganisms present on the skin that could potentially cause infection. If the skin is visibly soiled, it should be cleaned with soap and water before applying an alcohol-based chlorhexidine solution. Chlorhexidine is an effective antiseptic agent commonly used in healthcare settings for skin preparation due to its broad-spectrum antimicrobial properties.

# INFUSION NURSES SOCIETY (INS) STANDARDS

After applying the chlorhexidine solution, it's important to allow the puncture site to dry thoroughly before inserting the vascular access device. This helps ensure that the antiseptic solution has sufficient contact time to kill or inhibit any remaining microorganisms on the skin.

By adhering to these standards, healthcare professionals can significantly reduce the risk of bloodstream infections associated with vascular access procedures. This not only enhances patient safety but also contributes to the overall quality of care provided.

## Attempts

Grasping the INS (Infusion Nurses Society) standards regarding IV insertion attempts is crucial for optimizing patient comfort, treatment efficiency, and reducing potential complications.

# INFUSION NURSES SOCIETY (INS) STANDARDS

The INS standards recognize that IV insertion can be a significant source of stress for hospitalized patients, particularly for children. Therefore, the guidelines suggest limiting peripheral IV catheter (PIVC) insertion attempts to two per clinician. This limitation serves several important purposes:

## 1. Reducing Pain:

Multiple insertion attempts can cause increased discomfort for the patient due to repeated punctures. Limiting attempts helps minimize the pain experienced during the procedure.

## 2. Preventing Delay of Treatment:

Prolonged attempts at IV insertion can delay the start of necessary treatments or medications. By restricting attempts, healthcare providers can expedite the initiation of therapy, promoting timely patient care.

## 3. Preserving Veins:

Excessive attempts can lead to vein damage and compromise future access for IV therapy. Limiting the number of attempts helps preserve vein integrity, ensuring viable access for future procedures.

# INFUSION NURSES SOCIETY (INS) STANDARDS

### 4. Minimizing Complications:

Each insertion attempt carries the risk of complications such as bleeding, hematoma formation, or infection. By limiting attempts, healthcare providers can reduce the overall risk of procedural complications.

Additionally, if a clinician is unsuccessful after two attempts, the INS standards recommend involving a colleague with greater proficiency in PIVC insertion. This collaborative approach ensures that patients receive the highest quality of care from skilled healthcare professionals.

By adhering to these standards, healthcare providers can improve patient outcomes, enhance patient satisfaction, and promote safe and efficient IV therapy practices.

### Difficult Access

Comprehending the INS (Infusion Nurses Society) standards regarding difficult access is essential for delivering effective and compassionate healthcare, particularly in challenging scenarios.

# INFUSION NURSES SOCIETY (INS) STANDARDS

Difficult Intravenous Access (DIVA) occurs when multiple attempts to cannulate a vein are unsuccessful. This can be attributed to various factors such as the patient's age, underlying medical conditions, or a history of unsuccessful attempts. For instance, pediatric patients often have smaller veins, making them more challenging to access.

To address DIVA situations, the INS standards advocate for several strategies:

1. **Assigning IV Insertion to Skilled Nurses:**

Recognizing the importance of proficiency in IV insertion, the standards recommend assigning this task to nurses with demonstrated skill and experience. Skilled nurses are better equipped to navigate challenging situations and minimize patient discomfort.

2. **Utilizing Technology:**

The INS standards encourage the use of advanced technologies such as ultrasound or near-infrared light to improve the success rate of IV insertion. These technologies enable healthcare providers to visualize veins more clearly, facilitating accurate placement of the catheter even in difficult cases.

# INFUSION NURSES SOCIETY (INS) STANDARDS

By implementing these recommendations, healthcare providers can effectively manage DIVA situations, ensuring timely and successful IV access for patients. This approach not only enhances patient care but also reduces patient distress associated with multiple failed attempts. Ultimately, by adhering to these standards, healthcare professionals can uphold the principles of patient-centered care and optimize outcomes for individuals facing difficult intravenous access challenges.

# STUDY GUIDE

Welcome to the comprehensive study guide designed to accompany your workbook on starting peripheral intravenous (IV) lines. This guide is tailored to enhance your understanding and mastery of the essential skills required for successful IV insertion. By utilizing this resource, you'll develop confidence and proficiency in this critical aspect of healthcare practice.

<u>Section 1</u>: **Understanding Peripheral IV Insertion**

1.1. **Purpose and Importance:**

Define the purpose of peripheral IV insertion in healthcare settings.

Understand the significance of mastering this skill for patient care and treatment delivery.

1.2. **Anatomy and Physiology:**

Review the anatomy of veins and the physiology of blood circulation.

Identify key anatomical landmarks and vein characteristics relevant to IV insertion.

# STUDY GUIDE

1.3. **Indications and Contraindications:**

Learn the clinical indications for initiating peripheral IV therapy.

Understand the contraindications and factors influencing site selection for IV placement.

Section 2: **Preparation and Equipment**

2.1. **Gathering Supplies:**

Identify the necessary equipment and supplies for peripheral IV insertion.

Ensure proper organization and readiness of materials before initiating the procedure.

2.2. **Patient Assessment:**

Perform a comprehensive patient assessment to determine suitability for IV placement.

Consider factors such as medical history, allergies, and vascular status.

2.3. **Infection Control Measures:**

Implement appropriate hand hygiene and infection control protocols.

# STUDY GUIDE

Prepare the designated site using antimicrobial solutions and adhere to aseptic technique.

<u>Section 3:</u> **Peripheral IV Insertion Technique**

3.1. **Vein Selection and Assessment:**

Utilize tourniquets and other aids to facilitate vein identification and assessment.

Consider patient comfort and vein accessibility when selecting the insertion site.

3.2. **Catheter Insertion:**

Employ proper technique for stabilizing the vein and advancing the catheter.

Monitor for flashback and ensure appropriate catheter placement within the vein.

3.3. **Catheter Securing and Dressing:**

 - Secure the catheter in place using tape or securement devices.

Apply transparent dressings to maintain site integrity and minimize the risk of complications.

# STUDY GUIDE

Section 4: **Post-Insertion Care and Documentation**

**4.1. Flush and Assessment**:

Flush the IV catheter with saline solution to ensure patency.

Assess for adequate blood return and signs of infiltration or phlebitis.

4.2. **Patient Education:**

Provide thorough instructions to the patient regarding IV care and maintenance.

Address any concerns or questions related to the IV insertion procedure.

4.3. **Documentation:**

Document the details of the IV insertion procedure accurately and comprehensively.

Record the site, gauge, length of catheter, number of attempts, and patient response.

# STUDY GUIDE

**Conclusion:**

Congratulations on completing the comprehensive study guide on starting peripheral IVs. By mastering the skills and concepts outlined in this guide, you'll be well-equipped to perform IV insertion confidently and competently in clinical practice. Remember to practice diligently, prioritize patient safety, and seek guidance or support as needed. Good luck on your journey to becoming proficient in peripheral IV therapy.

# THANK YOU

As we come to the end of this workbook, remember that mastering the skill of starting peripheral IVs is a journey that requires dedication, practice, and ongoing learning. By following the steps outlined here and staying informed about the latest guidelines and best practices, you are equipped to provide safe and effective care to your patients.

Always prioritize patient safety and comfort, and never hesitate to seek assistance or ask questions if you encounter challenges along the way. Each IV insertion is an opportunity to make a positive impact on the lives of those in your care.

As you continue your healthcare journey, may you approach each IV insertion with confidence, skill, and compassion. Thank you for your commitment to excellence in vascular access, and may your efforts contribute to improved patient outcomes and experiences.

Keep learning, keep growing, and keep making a difference. Best wishes for success in all your future endeavors in healthcare.

Made in United States
Troutdale, OR
08/21/2024

22220478R00042